TEACHING VOLLEYING SKILLS

TO ELEMENTARY KIDS

A Simple
Developmental Pathway
to Success

David Olszewski
M. ED.

Print ISBN: 978-1-09831-233-6

eBook ISBN: 978-1-09831-234-3

INTRODUCTION

Teaching Volleying Skills to Elementary Age Students

Volleying Skills

Research shows that the acquisition of manipulative skills in the development of **Physical Literacy** increases the probability to continue active lifestyle habits and the participation in sport. In addition to this, the acquisition of **Manipulative Control** within the development of **Physical Literacy** is a reliable predictor of implementing and maintaining active lifestyles as adults Under a Movement Education Framework (MEF) volleying as a manipulative skill is considered one form of striking common to **Net and Wall Games** in the Games Area of curriculum. Other forms of striking skills include soccer kicking and heading, hockey propelling and sending, and batting and running. The text is simply dedicated to the process of *teaching volleying skills* basic to net and wall games at the elementary level and to show how to teach these skills taught within a basic and simple **Movement**

Education Framework Design (MEF). Successful volleying involves tracking and striking consistently and striking an object with different levels of force with the desired body part or manipulatives such rackets or paddles used to perform the skill. The games of " *Spike Ball and" Four Square* " often have more of a downward striking motion, it is important that this text is focused on volleying skills in more of an upward and forward motion and centered on those skills required to participated in **Net and Wall Games/Activities.** This design serves as a developmental movement guideline to assist in the process for every student to progress toward his or her own Physical Literacy regarding the ability successfully participate under the physical demands of the **Net and Wall** activities. The latest data shows that a large number Americans of various ages play some form of net and wall games whether in an instructional setting, interscholastic, recreational or leisure. (Reference the table on page 3 with approximate data) With this data in mind it is very apparent that net and wall sports can often carry over into adult hood as a part of the participation in active lifestyles and depending on the game itself potentially resulting in moderate to intense activity levels. Elementary age students experience the "Golden Age" of neuromuscular development. **Abels and Bridges** (2009) explain : " *In the primary years, students develop maturity and versatility in the use of fundamental motor skills that are further refined, combined and varied in the middle school years. These motor skills, now having evolved into specialized skills are used in increasingly complex movement environments in those middle school years." (NASPE 2004)*

Teaching children at this age to move skillfully in this form of sport only enhances their chances of pursuing more challenging experiences in net/wall sports as they progress in age. In any event giving students the necessary motor skills to move successfully is always a sound educational goal. **Abels and Bridges** also point out that "*Movement* (MEF) *is the heart/ core of any quality Physical Education Curriculum and is tied to Standard 1 and 2 of the current Shape America National Standards. Not only should we adhere to these standards but fulfill our responsibility as Physical Educators to teach our* *students this form of movement skill but as a valuable component in their pursuit of healthy and happy lifestyles."*

The Realities of the Gym/Programming

The challenging realities many of us Elementary Physical Educators face are usually focused on Adequate vs. Inadequate Space and scheduling limitations. Multipurpose spaces are the common for many elementary schools and with many doubling as cafeterias. This leads to scheduling limitations for adequate motor learning to take place in curriculum and often limiting Physical Education to once a week for 30 to 45 min. Although these challenges may certainly vary from community to community and state to state, it is appropriate to view this with the emphasis over the past years on increased classroom time and decreased specialists time that these challenges can be the norm rather than the exception. The goal of this book is to provide you with a clear and simple developmental design of teaching volleying skill within a movement progression to help each student experience success and challenge as they move forward in their abilities despite environmental and time limitations. This progression is based on a basic Movement Education Framework (MEF) designed to provide a simple understanding and implementation of the movement process of volleying through the elementary grades.

Physical Literacy
(Movement Development as a Process)

Physical Literacy is not a new term. As far back as the early twentieth century education scholars referred to physical literacy when describing beneficial elements related to educating the whole individual. The present definition (and some may vary slightly) is: " *A fundamental and valuable human capability that can be described as a disposition acquired by human individuals encompassing the motivation, confidence, physical competence, knowledge and understanding that establishes purposeful physical pursuits as an integral part of their lifestyle*". Kriellaars explains that "fitness is an outcome of physical literacy not visa versa"(2017). He cites the benefits of physical literacy; creative thinking through free play, emotion and social development, the enhancement physical motor skill, increased cognitive processing and increased physical fitness to name a few. He goes further to explain that physical literacy is" building a movement vocabulary " I look at

Physical Literacy as the complete package of physical motor experiences that enhance an individual's propensity to move well and move often, thus enhancing a healthy lifestyle. Ireland Great Britain and Canada have used this as a guiding to Physical Education. As Pointed out in an article by " Coaching Ireland " (2017) **Physical Literacy does not happen by accident: "** it takes a combined effort from parents, schools, community recreation and sport. It is a complex process and requires careful planning and quality delivery." Teaching within a Movement Education Framework (MEF) is a perfect developmental guide to building physical literacy in our students and following that framework is key to them acquiring to successful acquisition.

CHAPTER 1

Movement Education Framework (MEF A Simple Understanding."Bridges and Abels explain that Movement Education's roots evolved primarily from Rudolph Laban (1879 – 1958) who studied the elements of movement and how they related to dance. Laban was mostly focused on the effort (speed and force the body applies when moving) as related to dance and specifically how the body communicates and expresses itself through movement. Stanley (1977) and Logdson with colleagues (1984) developed a framework of movement from Laban's concepts and applied it to Physical Education Curriculum and Physical Literacy basic to all areas of human movement and activity. Unfortunately **Abels and Bridges** explain: that the approach to movement education " *became more and more complex"* due to disagreements from a variety of theorists on how to approach Movement Education Framework. As a result by the 1990's the approach was confusing and often intimidating in a practical setting. MEF lost a great deal of momentum it received in the 1960's 70's and 80's. As an undergraduate I was educated and trained in the Movement Education process as a Physical Educator at Bridgewater State College (which is now Bridgewater State University) and I have never strayed from a Movement Education approach. From my experiences these movement concepts and principals are sound and extremely beneficial in the development process of developing and enhancing Physical Literacy in our students. Just approach it from a simple and basic understanding! So now let's look at how Logsdon applied these movement concepts a broad based way to the three learning domains.

(Blooms Taxonomy) To understand how our students learn we must understand how the brain learns. Blooms Taxonomy guides us in that.

- Cognitve (Understanding and Knowledge)

- Psychomotor (Body Movement and Skills)

- Affective (Emotions, Feelings , Social Behavior)

Logsdon and Stanley took four concepts of movement and applied these to Physical Education.

- Body (What body does)

- Space (Where the body goes)

- Effort (Speed and Force the Body Uses)

Relationship (What and Who the Body Relates to)

Logsdon then identified three areas of curriculum to teach, maintain and enhance Physical Literacy in all aspects basic to human movement in active lifestyles.

1. Games/Sport

2. Dance

3. Gymnastics

Although my curriculum primarily focuses on Dance and Games, and some Gymnastics. (Gymnastics is minimal due to space and equipment constraints) My hat goes off to those Physical Educators who can implement all three areas of curriculum to their students equally as they are able balance and address the Physical Literacy needs of their students.

As mentioned earlier, this book is specifically focused on volleying skills related to Net/Wall Games which is just one area of Games/Sport Movement. A complete movement framework is vast and detailed because as we increase our movement language and physical literacy we encounter many development tasks and aspects we need learn and experience in a Physical Education environment to gain competency and/or proficiency in all areas of movement. This may not be as realistic as we would like it be to when only being able to see students on a limited basis for limited times in limited space. It's my belief that despite these limitations, a simple and basic understanding movement needs in children will benefit our students greatly in their motor development and Physical Literacy. I should know. I have taught for 32 years encountering these limitations, yet my student's progress in their physical capabilities each and every lesson. Let me show you how.

Differentiating for Success

Differentiation is nothing new to developmental Physical Education. Teachers teaching with developmentally sound practice methods have been doing it for years. Physical Educators have differentiated the activities/tasks that they present to students so that each student can progress forward in his/her abilities while accepting and confronting new movement challenges related to the lesson/unit he is learning. The best example of this is what Muska Moston (1984) explained when discussing teaching styles for success in Physical Education. He posed the question this way: *If you had high jump a bar that you wanted your students to jump over, How could you assure that every student was successful at it and at the same time move forward in his/her abilities?* **After some discussion, Moston simply angled the bar from low to high**. That is a simple example of differentiating to individual abilities. Every student is capable of jumping over the bar at a different ability level and yet is free to make decisions as to what height they can confront for a greater challenge. Giving students decisions in their movement challenges can be applied to various sports and games movement experiences for elementary students. Successful experiences can also lead to greater confidence when confronting new challenges. For example: The student who catches a balloon or the student who can catch a bean bag of greater challenge are both catching successfully. Is the skill of catching being taught? Of course! One just learns at a different ability level and needs to track slower and with proper teacher guidance and decision making will hopefully progress forward over time tracking faster and catching with more complexity and refined skill. The operative phrase is "Success Through Differentiation." In other words, teach to each individual's ability and keep the bar angled and make available developmentally appropriate equipment for each student to experience success and greater challenge, Another example could be during throwing and catching partner skills, you make yarn balls and wiffle balls available to various ability levels so that each student can track at different speeds and catch by grabbing onto to something of softer or harder texture.

Why MEF? Think of It This Way!

As mentioned earlier Movement Education is not a new idea. It has been a significant part of Physical Education dating back to the 1960's but unfortunately it's practical application was implemented with some confusion and ineffectiveness. So again, let's keep it simple! Take these movement concepts and examine a movement skill. Say you are teaching basketball dribbling skills to third graders. Look about gym and think of it this way.

Body - What is the Body Doing ? = Dribbling a Basketball

Space – Where is the Body Going? = Personal and General Space

Effort – What speed or force is the body using = Probably medium speed and medium force over the ball for control.

Relationship – What and Who are your students relating to? = The ball, the ground, other students.

It's simple! All of these four concepts are occurring at some time in the movement of your students. Now ask yourself this question? What is the main emphasis of the experience? *Probably dribbling the basketball in control, Right!* That would be the **Body Concept**! Now take it a step forward and think of the other concepts. Is there anything else in any of the other concepts that stands out or needs correcting. *Maybe some kids need to dribble softer with less* **Effort** *or some using personal* **Space** *rather than moving throughout in general* **Space.** *Are they* **Relating** *to the ball they are using or should they change to another that is more appropriate for their movement ability. Maybe they need something less or more challenging to improve.* Your main emphasis was the **Body** movement of dribbling. Keeping in mind those other areas you observe through your own movement analysis offers you a developmental guide for keeping your experience successful and challenging enough for each student to move forward by touching on other concepts if the need is there. Let's use another example: In this lesson I emphasize two concepts. I am teaching soccer passing lesson to second grade students. One of my teaching cues is" Make your partner a good receiver and passer, " Pass it so your partner can get it back to you."! My major learning concept is on **Relationships.** Will each student work skillfully and cooperatively a partner. My other emphasis is on **Body.** Students pass the ball with the inside of the foot and receive the ball in control with the foot.

Guess What! All four concepts are involved. But I mainly focused on two concepts, **Relationships** and the **Body.** Let's take a look at the other two. **Effort –** Students had to pass at the right speed for control. **Space –** Students had to maintain an open play space where they could play without interfering with others. Maybe you would have taught the lesson by emphasizing the **Space** concept. If the need was there, maybe students in the class would have to practice controlling their ball in open space better before moving forward as a partner or team player. Where the need is, emphasize the concept or concepts. See! It's that simple. Even without referring to a Movement Education Framework (MEF) we tend to use our understanding of what students are capable of physically to teach age appropriate tasks/activities. Referencing a Movement Education Framework adds to that developmental movement understanding and gives us a simple and basic developmental guide for meeting the movement needs of our students. *Langton and Baumgarten* explain: " **Body,**

Space, Effort and Relationship - *the four aspects of Laban's movement framework – offer a useful structure for organizing elementary physical education lessons.* " They go further to identify four core values of teaching curriculum within a movement framework.

- **Use a Movement Framework as a basis for curriculum content in games, gymnastics and dance.**

- **Blend health enhancing physical activity and physical fitness concepts into all lessons.**

- **Provide exemplary instruction and assessment in order to make learning meaningful, challenging, enjoyable and enduring.**

- **Create and maintain a learning environment that encourages students to be the best they can be through hard work and continual self- improvement.**

Each Movement Concept Has Some Theme

Simply put, each Movement Concept has some movement themes. A theme is simply and area of movement development that helps you target movement skills better. Because volleying skills are games related and we are specifically targeting volleying as a manipulative skill I will present the games area in curriculum with a basic view of the themes within each Movement Concept Area in our Movement Education Framework (MEF). The back of the book shows a more detailed version. I am presenting this as a more simplified version that is easy to implement.

Body (What the Body Does In Games) *Manipulative Actions* - striking, kicking, throwing, catching, dribbling, propelling.

Space (Where the body goes) - Personal Space, General Space.

Effort (How much force/speed you are applying to the Skill) – Fast , slow , hard and soft.

Relationships (What are you relating to during the skill) – people, Object, Equipment.

Teaching Movement with Purpose and Movement for Competency/ Proficiency.

When describing their " Application of Findings" Shape America describes it this way:

"Shape America considers the development of motor skill competence to be the highest priority in grade level outcomes. As research has shown , skill competency is essential for student engagement, intrinsic motivation, perceived competency, participation in physical activity and subsequently, sufficient levels of health related fitness" Because movement is the **Core** of Physical Education curriculum, " Shape America has targeted a core base of Movement Skills to be taught as outcomes of achievement for every student to possess in the area of Physical Literacy so that the Physically Literate student will possess a greater potential to participate in healthy, active lifestyles. Among these outcomes are the manipulative skills of **Volleying Overhand, Volleying Underhand (with hands and arms)** and **Volleying with a Short and Long Implement.** When teaching any movement experience I always consider how that experience relates to human activity as a person grows,

develops and becomes competent. Movementexperiences, whether they are tasks of progression or activities designed to enhance movement skills in a successful yet challenging enough environment for everyone (**differentiation**) should have a core purpose. *Judith Rink (2012)* gives an example of an Elementary Physical Education Program with purpose. "***The second grade class will work at combining locomotor patterns by practicing separately and then develop a routine of movement by the end of the lesson. The teacher will focus on (Blooms Taxonomy) cognitive, psychomotor and affective objectives.***" This is a defensible and sound practice. *Rink (2012)* then gives an example of an non defensible program without movement purpose.

"***The second grade class really likes to play the parachute, that is what the second grade classes will do all day. The teacher writes all of the fun things they like to do with the parachute and the teacher writes them down and implements them.*** I often refer to this approach as "*Random Acts of Activity!*" If we follow a basic movement framework for our students then we will be able to recognize the meaningful connection to the movement challenges and progressions that our students accomplish as they experience a connection to movement basic to human activity (Physical Literacy). Essentially we are bringing the curriculum to our students! Not the one size fits all, but rather a developmental process that allows students to achieve and progress. A basic example that I'm sure many of us are familiar with is soccer player who dribbles and kicks the ball and explores it with various parts of the foot in personal and general space. Once control is established with competence he/she begins to share it with various passing skills in open space. When this is established then he/

she begins to move and pass and keep away from others to partners or teammates in progressively larger groups. As concepts and skills improve he/she begins to play invasion like games with more complexity in the game that require more **skill,**(Psychomotor) **strategy/tactics** (Cognitive) and **teamwork** (Affective). It is certainly my goal and probably the goal of most Physical Educators that joy of movement in games, dance and gymnastics exists in every learning experience my students participate in. To me it is a simple formula! If you are providing an environment that allows for success and progress in movement skill and developmental growth under a movement framework, the enjoyment of moving well should be always there, whether it is a 3 vs 3 soccer game or performing a dance individually or in groups or playing tag with different levels of dodging skill and speed. Activity for the sake of activity may deny our students the necessary motor skills they need to become Physically Literate. Movement Experiences and Activities with purpose is what we should always strive for, so we can give our students the necessary movement skills basic to human activity.

CHAPTER 2

Teaching to Every Student

Let's Go Back to Motor Learning 101 .....!

As mentioned earlier, Movement Development is a process. When students are competent and successful in movement experiences they are more likely to continue to be active. Competence or Proficiency = Greater Activity! As we teach within a simple and basic movement framework, maintaining an understanding of developmental motor stages children experience is vital when implementing a movement curriculum that is geared towards individualized success and growth. So let us review the three phases of **Motor Learning** individuals go through when learning motor tasks/ activities. First, let's understand what learning truly is. *Rink* explains that **Learning** is thought of as a "relatively permanent change in behavior resulting from experiences and training and interacting with biological processes." She points out that one of the problems teachers face in directing learning processes and in assessing, is that learning cannot be directly observed! Learning can only be observed through a individuals performance. Performance is observable, but learning is not! Because motor performance is what we observe as teachers to indicate how well children learn in a physically active environment, it is ever more important that kids move with competence and success in their paths to physically literate/ physically active lifestyles.

Cognitive Phase

The learner is heavily focused on how the movement be performed for success. At his phase visual demonstration is extremely valuable to the learner. The learner involves himself in extensive concentration when performing the skill/task. *Note: It is important not to give too much information to the learner at this phase so he or she is not overwhelmed. An example could be giving the learner a task of kicking the soccer ball with various parts of your foot into open space in the gym, bringing the foot back and kicking it. Characteristics of this phase:*

- Thought processes are heavily involved (Concentration)

- The learner is not able to attend to small details in the task.

Associative Phase

During this phase the learner is capable of concentrating more on the dynamics of the skill, focusing on timing and more refined, smooth and efficient actions. The learner becomes more capable of attending to various components of the skill. A learner may spend quite a bit of time in this phase of motor learning. *Note: An example may be the soccer player who works at specifically contacts the ball when passing it with the inside of the foot while stiffening up the ankle repeatedly sending the ball to a teammate while controlling the ball by moving through space. Characteristics of this phase:*

- The learner can begin to focus on the refinement of the skill.

- The learner benefits from feedback

- The learner can start to cope with the external demands of the environment around him or her as they gain skill in the task/activity and does not always have to concentrate on the skill.

Automatic Phase

This is the phase where the learner does not have to concentrate on the skill. The skill now becomes an automatic movement, where the learner can attend to other stimulus around him. *Note: An example could be the skilled soccer player who doesn't have to concentrate at shooting the ball into the goal, but rather dribbling around the defender as his or she approaches the goal. Characteristics of this phase:*

- The skill performed is more automatic. The learner does not have to attend to the skill itself.

- The performance has consistency to it and the learner is constantly capable of adapting to changing demands in his/her environment.

By looking at these phases, it is apparent that children experience different motor stages when learning a skill. To get to one phase, they have to experience the previous one to progress forward. When teaching our students, we see that each student experiences these phases at different time periods for differing durations. A student may have to spend longer periods of time in the cognitive phase prior to progressing to the associative phase.

Another student may progress more rapidly and need to encounter greater movement challenges as he or she progresses through the associative phase into the automatic phase. Every student has different motor abilities and needs based on their mental and physical (neuromuscular) development. The need for differentiation becomes apparent.

Tips for Sound Practice "Approaching Every Lesson for Everyone to Learn and Progress !"

Maximize Participation

Without moving and moving often, physical skill cannot be obtained in a reasonable time frame.

Years ago during my undergraduate work at Bridgewater State University, A professor used this analogy to support the approach of maximizing participation in Physical Education class:" *If a classroom teacher is teaching literacy he or she would not have 20 students share 4 pencils.*" Each student needs a pencil to learn and practice for a significant time period! The same is true for Physical Education. For physical literacy to be developed, we must recognize that Movement Development is a process and movement experiences should be maximized so that each student has adequate time on task to practice and progress forward. A bean bag for every student learning to catch! A soccer ball for every student learning to dribble and so on! This is particularly true if we refer to those Motor learning Phases students experience. This can certainly be said of the **Cognitive Phase** when each student must concentrate on the object they have and practice when developing a manipulative skill. Couple this with those programs that are only once a week, it is vital that a teacher provides optimal movement time for each student to develop. When examining Sound Practice I like to adhere to these three Principles. Is each student:

1. *Active Enough*

2. *Successful Enough*

3. *Challenged Enough*

To progress forward.

Active Learning Time and Movement Time

Active learning time is that time in each class that students are engaged in learning. Think of this. When your students are engaged in performing the task or activity, listening and processing your instruction, debriefing or watching other students demonstrate, they are engaged in active learning. In other words learning is not just taking place by movement but those other areas within a lesson to further their learning. If students are engaged in active learning over 80 % of the class, that's a lot of learning! Certainly we all strive for 100%, but class dynamics tend to vary from class to class and the possible need to attend to any classroom organization and/or management need certainly may exist. *Movement time* is that time critical to each student acquiring skill and progressing forward. Keeping every student engaged in performing the movement focus of the lesson over 60% of the time is certainly acceptable and worthy to strive for. Students need to move for the vast majority of the lesson to progress. Hence the need for *Clear, Brief, and Concise Instruction* so we can get our students moving. In other words **" Keep your Students Busy and Learning".**

Remember Differentiation "Angle the Bar for Learning"

Remember **Moston's** analogy. If all students can successfully perform at their own abilities, then we allow them to successfully progress forward through their own successes. *Abel* explains that: " *providing choices enhances learning,,,the challenge is to provide extensions of the movement by making it more or less challenging* for success *as compared to a traditional approach.* I referred earlier to two students who were performing catching skills as they learned to track an object out of the air and catch it with their hands and fingers before it hits the ground. One student requires a balloon for success and the other student a bean bag. Both were given choices to achieve the skill. Both are successful and will be encouraged through their own motivations when they are ready or with guidance from the teacher to move into greater challenges as they progress in their movement literacy. On the other hand, a traditional approach would be that everyone is given the same ball despite his/her ability, opening up the potential for a number of students to fail in the task. This is not to say that failure is not a part of learning, but keeping students successful increases their potential to progress continually. Remember *Differentiate*.

Objects that Allow for Differentiation.

Meeting the students as to where their needs exist as described previously is a key component of differentiation. Essentially bringing the curriculum to them allows for vertical development in these volleying skill experiences. I have always taught by presenting objects of varying weight and size that allow students to track and volley with greater success as they progress vertically. The pictures display objects that I have used that are offered in each student's developmental path toward greater success and challenge. You may find there is a general range of objects used at various grade levels that allow enough variance for a variety of needs related to tracking and tapping/volleying , although in some cases you may progress forward a bit beyond that object range if the needs are there. **Note:** *This ball/object range is based on objects that I have found to enhance success and progress. By no means is this range set in stone but rather offered as a developmentally progressive guide.*

Your own creative Innovations may lead to an object that enhances success. You never know!

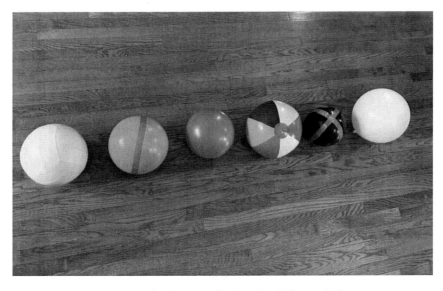

Developmental range for grades K through five.

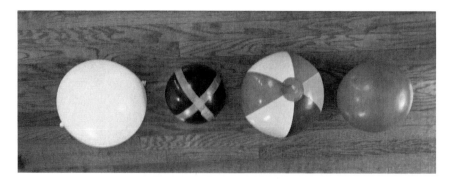

Suggested object range for primary age students.

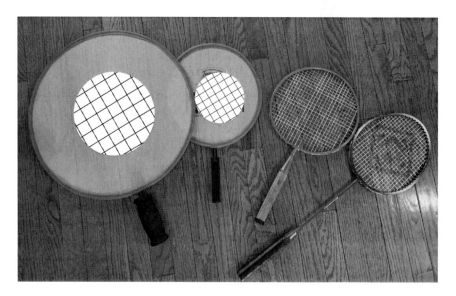

Racket range for grades K through five.

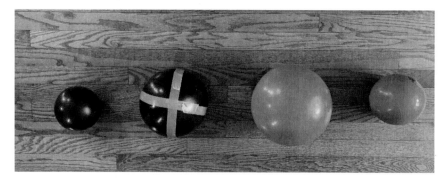

Object range for racket volleying " Grades K through five.

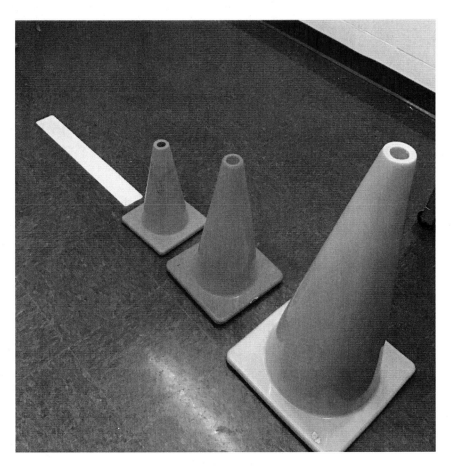

Obstacle Height Progression as K Through five students progress toward net play.***

Remember to Teach within a Developmental Movement Framework.

Teaching within a Movement Education Framework (MEF) offers the teacher a movement guide which is appropriate for the developmental movement needs of each student which are basic to human activity and physical literacy. When we target those developmental needs with appropriate movement tasks or activities we set each student on the right course of progression. Remember if our students are successful and competent, chances are certainly greater for them to participate further and extend themselves in their movement abilities. Through competence or proficiency (in this case regarding manipulative skills) comes the greater potential to experience healthy, active lifestyles.

Designing and Environment for Learning

A teaching environment may change depending on the movement needs of the class. *Ring* explains : " *One of the first problems with using the descriptions of skills found in many text books as a guide for teaching a skill is that the skill will look different if it is adapted to different environments.*" A soccer dribble will look different if you are closely guarded as opposed to dribbling freely without any defender upon you. You may have to keep the ball close to you with a defender, but not as close to you if you are dribbling up field unguarded. In other words a skill that is practiced at the *cognitive level* may need a **closed environment** (environment that remains the same and predictable without out any stimulus that would interfere with the practicing of the skill) . An example would be a student practicing tapping a balloon upward in person space with either hand and trying to keep it off the ground. As this student progresses in skill, the environment may change as they encounter sharing taps with a partner. The environment is now an **open environment**. (The environment the two students are participating in has more unpredictability) The student(s) have to react to the balloon coming to them while attempting to send back to his or her partner. This environment can be ever changing and requires the student to adapt successfully as he or she continues to progress forward. We will see this in the volleying lessons progression presented in the next section.

CHAPTER 3

Assessment

Assessment is simply collecting data and measuring what is learned by your student(s). Assessment as explained in this text is not presented as extensive and detailed, but rather to provide a basic format of strategies that can be used and a spring board for engaging in other forms seen as effective for the teacher. I personally find assessment as an effective means of self - assessing my own delivery of content to my classes as well as how well students are learning. Because of the various scheduling challenges many of us face as Physical Educators, I view assessment as being implemented in a timely and concise manner, making sure that it is not time consuming but rather appropriate for what the teacher is looking for in the movement development of each student. Remember, many of us are extremely limited in the time we see our students and oft experience back to back classes with only a few minutes between that may be three or four grades apart. An example could be that you may have a 2nd grade followed by a 5th grade class a few minutes later. ***Schiemer explains: "Not surprisingly, elementary physical education specialists find they have very little teaching time available. According to calculations (Kelly 1989) practitioners who meet students once a week for a 30 minute class have 8.1 hours actual learning time for the entire school year – the actual time available to the student for on-task practice.*** Based on evidence like this, I would caution anyone with scheduling limitations to not let assessment consume your program but rather use it as an effective and time efficient tool that measures learning.

Formative Assessment

This form of Assessment simply measures the progress of the individual(s) performance during classes/units throughout the duration. An example could be a 2nd grade class in basketball skills : *Measuring each students progress during the lesson of " Basket Ball Dribbling " Are they providing the right amount of force over the ball to control it to themselves?*

Summative Assessment

This form of assessment simply measures the progress of the individuals(s) performance at the conclusion of a class/unit. An example could a 3rd grade lesson in throwing and receiving: *" each student is performing an overhand throw by stepping forward with his or her opposite foot and twisting the waist as the arm moves forward in the direction of their partner by the end of a 4 lesson unit".*

Qualitative Assessment

This form of assessment measures the quality of the movement skill/performance and involves knowledgeable movement analysis methods from the teacher. Some examples could be:

When your performed a basketball foul shot from the foul line, was your elbow in and your dominant hand placed behind the ball as you pushed it at the basket?

When you made your over hand throw did your hand pass your ear and did you twist your waist and follow through.

Does your dance transition in to three changing shapes throughout   your routine?

Quantitative Assessment

This form of assessment measures the quantity of the skill(s) being performed. The intent being that the more often the skill is performed the increase in performance ability. Some examples could be:

- How many balloon taps can you make to your partner using your hands by not letting the balloon hit the ground?

- How many bowling pins did you knock down by sliding your beanbags at the pins in two tries?

- How many throws and catches did you make to your partner in the lesson?

- How many passes did your team make in 3 & 3 basketball keep away.

Authentic Assessment

This form of assessment is also referred to as an **Alternative Assessment** and refers to the skills and decisions the student typically faces in performance/game/activity situations. This may require a higher order of thinking and reflection the environment and performance. Assessment practices may vary regarding this form as opposed to more traditional assessment. One can argue that both have a purpose and place in a developmentally progressive program. **Schiemer points out: " In Physical Education, developmentally appropriate authentic or alternative assessment results in teacher decisions based primarily on ongoing individual assessment in children as they participate in physical education class** *activities (formative evaluation), not only on test scores (summative evaluation) (Graham 1992). A student should progress in their psychomotor, affective and cognitive domains, developing positive skills, attitudes and knowledge about physical education."* Examples can be:

- In a 4&4 keep away soccer game, are you moving to open space consistently to receive a pass when your team has the ball? Were you communicating to your teammates in a productive and positive manor?

- Is your paddle consistently in a ready and striking position to receive a hit from your partner or opposing player across the net?

- Are you seeing where you are going when while dribbling the floor hockey ball into open space during a stealing and dribbling challenge with classmates?

- During two base cricket ,as a fielder are you looking consistently to throw to the correct base that your partner is covering to get the runner out as the best strategy.

As you will soon see that when you read through grade level progressions, you will notice that at the end of each lesson progression, I have included a basic assessment statement framed as a guide in targeting the movement skills pertaining to that particular developmental progression. This can be offered as a spring board to engage in other forms of assessment the teacher uses as a valuable tool of measurement. These forms of assessment may include:

- **Peer Review** - Students modeling to visually demonstrate correct movement content (quality) of the lesson as well as positive affective and cognitive qualities.

- **Individual, partner or team/group reflection** – Students reflect and report on elements of success psychomotor, affective and cognitive.

- **Journals** – Reflecting on individual, group of team performance psychomotor, affective and cognitive.

- **Drawings, Sketches or Pictures** – Reflecting the correct skill performed in the lesson or lessons.

- **Measuring the quantity of the performance** - How often are the tasks/skills successfully performed?

CHAPTER 4

Lessons that Teach Volley Skills

When looking at volleying, it is apparent that volleying is mostly an upward motion as it relates to net and wall games. Children need to learn how to track an object and contact it consistently as they send it directly ahead or upward with a manipulative, one hand or both hands . A tennis player sends the ball over the net in an upward " C " swing , contacting it for top spin as it goes over the net. A volleyball player is constantly positioning himself under the ball to contact it upward with forearms or hands and/or fingers. A badminton player positions themselves to contact the ball with the racket often slashing it up and over with clear contact. Even if you are looking and racket ball, pickle ball or handball, the motion is often upward within the mechanics of the skill to drive the ball forward. Obviously the exception to this is when the environment warrants an overhead downward strike such as a volleyball spike or an overhand tennis or badminton smash. This text is dedicated to those frequent volleying skills that must precede those highly competitive over hand downward skills often used in highly competitive game environments. The lessons presented in this text encompass grades K to the very onset of grade five. These lessons progress under a **Developmental Movement Education Framework.** When looking at how students to progress. *Rink (2014) explains:" When a teacher develops progressions for teaching skills from simple to more complex, the teacher is hoping that there will be a transfer from one level of ability to another". She goes on to say:" Teachers can determine if their progressions are successful by determining the extent to which practice in one* *situation transfers to the other,"* The Movement Experiences show a progression from general exploration to more refined and specific tasks as students would developmentally progress forward in their motor skill and confront the more complex demands of the environments they are participating in. Although many of the units are 3 to 5 lessons, this may certainly vary in length due to the practice time students need to progress forward as determined by the teacher. It is also important to note that at the beginning of each lesson there is included a **warm – up review which emphasizes body memory.** To re – experience the skills applied to the previous lesson is important to each student for **body memory purposes** and the ability to progress forward. This is particularly necessary for those programs that may only offer Physical Education once per week with a week or so between lessons.

Objects Used to Teaching Volley Skills at the Primary Age Level.

Because the movement focus in on each student tracking and striking successfully while being able to confront greater challenges and challenging environments, allowing for each student to participate with an object appropriate to his or her tracking and striking needs is ***critical for success***. Meeting the student as to where there needs are is important. Essentially bringing the curriculum to them. Using a variety of appropriate development objects targets the students developmental need. Does the object bounce or stay in flight long enough to be tracked is the object large enough to contact consistently as they transfer their learning experiences and progress vertically. Allowing a variety of developmentally appropriate objects to be available in the primary years for each lesson can be equipment intensive, but objects such as balloons, beach balls and light plastic balls are very cost efficient! Each student is climbing the ladder of ability based on teacher guided or student driven choices.

These choices should be made based on weight, size and speed of flight. As an example: Your class may have a diverse range of track abilities. Having beach balls, balloons with one or two strips of tape around them for greater weight and of course a regular balloon are all appropriate for those diverse tracking needs. Maybe Johnny or Heather are not ready to progress to a beach ball from a balloon, but need a transitional object such as a tapped balloon for greater weight, challenge and success before transitioning to a beach ball. When *Rink (2012)* explains the **"Transfer of Learning"** process during the teaching of skills: *" **Bilateral Transfer** " is when you learn how to alternate hands when dribbling in basketball. **Intertask Transfer** You learn one skill and it transfers to another, like from tennis to racquetball. **Intratask Transfer** is when you practice a skill from one condition and it transfers that skill to another condition. An example of this is a successful volleyball set moving from a trainer to a volleyball.*

The variance of suitable objects for volleying enhances the success of students through grade levels as they experience the three learning areas presented, particularly **Intratask Transfer.**

The Process of the Units and Lessons Presented

The basic purpose of the movement experiences presented in this text is to show a developmental movement process of tracking and striking (volleying skills) while showing the process of movement from simple to more complex skills. Presented to you are units that encompass those volleying experiences common to all forms **net / wall games** that include volleying skills. These units are broken down into 3 - 5 lesson experiences, but may not have to be fixed as a one lesson experience. As an example, if you are looking at *lesson two* **Grade 1** movement experiences, it may take some class's two lessons to achieve the competency required to move forward and you certainly may not get through all the learning experiences in one lesson. That is certainly appropriate for whatever the developmental needs of individuals or classes in general require to volleying skill. In fact although the experiences are grade level based, a teacher could find the movement experiences from a previous grade appropriate for the next grade level or possibly or visa versa. Again it all depends on the motor skills and needs of the class make up. You will also notice a brief review for body memory at the beginning of each new experience. This is especially beneficial for those programs being taught once a week.

What You Can Take from the Lesson/ Unit Process.

Depending on how often you see your students ,you may decide to follow this process of learning experiences in detail as a developmental guide to enhancing the volleying process of each student.

You may decide to generalize your approach and bypass or blend some experiences together.

You may decide to review the same experiences to reinforce movement skill as a vehicle to successfully progress forward.

You may decide to provide frequent class activity based experiences as a means of reinforcing volleying skill. *As noted earlier, volleying skills should be successfully experienced and taught prior implementing this approach so that each student can experience a high range of success.*

You may find that some classes or students may progress at a faster rate of success and actually participate at a higher grade level experience. *It is important to note, that although these experiences are presented as grade learning experiences, they are developmentally based and should offer an environment that is appropriate for each student to progress. Differentiating to students or class needs in general is always a good practice. Remember " Angle the Bar for Success " (Moston)*

A teachers ability to provide appropriate learning experiences through his or her own movement analysis of each student is key to their growth and success. In addition to this a sound strategy you may not see in the unit/lesson progressions but should be applied commonly is.

1. **Student or students demonstrating (student modeling) to present a visual picture of correct mechanics and play.**

CHAPTER 5

Unit Plans

Kindergarten

· ·

Striking with different body parts including arms and hands.

Equipment – balloons and lite inflatable balls and beach balls.

Body - striking with hands and arms emphasis

Space – personal , general, high , medium, and low

Effort - various of speeds over object

Relationship – to floor space, wall space

· ·

1A Find a ball or balloon of your choice. Let's begin to strike with different body parts. Can you strike your object in different ways with your hands... your arms .....legs.....feet.....head.

1B Keep your eye on your object and watch that body part strike it into space. Remember to always look for and open space to strike to. It can be a close space or an open space away from you. Think of many different ways to strike with those body parts.....hands.....arms.....legs....feet....head. (Exploration is open ended. Students may strike of the ground, out of the air or on the bounce.)

1C Now let's explore our hands and arms as we strike our object. Remember to think of different ways to use them to strike with. Are your hands closed when you strike or are they open when you strike? Feel what it is like to strike with an open hand sometimes and a closed hand other times. Remember to watch your hand or hands strike your object into open space.

1D Remember, You can strike it down, ahead or up into the air.

1E How did it feel to strike with your hands when they were open and when they were closed. Did you notice where you ball went after you tapped it.

1F Now let's explore our arms and strike your object with different parts of your arms into open space, What parts of your arms are you striking with and what does it feel like ?

2A From last lesson let's review by striking your object in different ways with our hands and arms into open spaces. Do you remember that your hands can be open or closed? What part of your arms are you striking with?

2B Start to explore striking your object with two hands sometimes and two arms sometimes. Can you feel the difference between using both arms and both hands compared to one hand and one arm.

2C Now let's try both ways to strike with your arms and hands. When I say strike with …. One hand……two hands….one arm…… both arms and remember to try to always send your object into open space.

2D Let's begin to explore striking our object with our hands and arms into space by making it go up and into the air more. Remember to keep your eye on the object when you strike it with your hands or arms under or behind it.

2E Can you strike the object goes up to yourself up into other open spaces. Where are your hands or arms when contacting your object.

2F This time when you strike you object, see if your hands and arms can go under it or behind it as you strike it.

Striking Objects with a Paddle

• •

Equipment - short paddles, balloons tapped and without tape, beach balls and inflatable balls of different sizes.

Body - striking an object with an implement. One or two hands gripping the implement at handle.

Space – high , medium , low , personal and general.

Effort – Applying various levels of speed (force) over the object.

Relationship – To paddle , objects, floor and wall.

• •

1A Find a paddle and shake hands with the handle. Hold it with your hand and wrap your fingers around it. Pretend that you are striking at an object and swing that paddle forward in different ways. Maybe from over head ...your side.. and under your waist.

1B Now try gripping your paddle with one or two hands and feel what it is like to swing your paddle forward from those same areas of your body....over....side... and under.

1C This time find an object and start to strike it with the big flat part of the paddle. We call that the face. See how often you can strike your object with one or two hands with the face of your paddle. What parts of your body are you striking it from.

Remember, maybe you will strike from over.....side...or under. (Keep in mind that students may tap their object on the ground, bounce, or in the air).

1D Now on my command strike from your side....strike from over your head....strike from under your waist. Remember to keep your eye on your object as you strike.

1E Let's keep striking it, but this time concentrate on send your object into open spaces as often as you can. You might strike it to a close open space or far into big open spaces away from you.

> **Assessment – *Measuring that students are striking the object on the face of the paddle consistently and into general and personal open space.***

2A Let's strike the object with our paddle on the face of the paddle like we did last lesson. Keep your eye on the object and strike. Remember to keep your strike close to you in space or away from you in space. Don't forget those areas of the body.

2B This time let's start to play " Tap it Close " . Feel what it is like to tap your object close to you as often as you can. Can you keep the object with you as you tap.

2C Let's play : Tap Count ". Count how many taps you can do to yourself. (Remember taps can be from the ground, air or on the bounce for successful tracking).

2D Let's share our object with a partner by tapping it from the ground and back to your partner. Make your partner a good player by tapping the object back to them. Remember keep you r eye on your object and try to strike it with the face of the paddle.

2E Find a new partner and see how you do. Go wherever the object goes and strike it back to your partner.

> **Assessment – Measuring that students are striking with the face of the paddle from different areas of the body into personal space individually and to a partner.**

Grade One Lessons

Volleying Using Your Hands and Arms,

First Grade Hand Striking

Unit

* Represents Main Focus . Other areas listed represent the Side Emphasis of the Lesson or Lessons presented.

. . . .

Equipment- Lite Weight Balls, Balloons for differentiation of various movement needs for tracking and striking.

Objective – Each student strikes an object with hands and arms in various ways.

Body - Striking with hands away and to self, upward and downward

Space - Striking with hands into personal open space or general open space.

Relationship – Floor space , air space and wall space, sometimes to a partner

Effort – Various levels of force over the object

. . . .

Learning Experiences **Note** – although not included in the lesson experiences, having students model for class briefly is valuable visual feedback for students.

1 A *Strike your ball or balloon with one or two hands or your arms into open space. Keep your eye on the object and watch it hit your arms or hands.*

1B *Now see how many different open spaces you can strike to. Keep your eye on the ball when striking. Remember, eye on object and strike with hands or lower arms.*

1 C *Now that you have struck it in different ways, start striking your object upward or down ward or ahead more with you hand/ hands or arms contacting the object.*

1 D *Continue striking your object upward, forward or down-ward using the open air, floor or wall space you see.*

1E *Practice striking your object by tapping it into close spaces sometimes and striking it away into farther away spaces. Feel the difference between a close tap and a faraway strike. Remember to use your lower arms and hands. How do your arms and hands move when you tap closer compared to when you strike away?*

Assessment - Measuring that students are contacting the object with hands and lower arms at different levels.

2A *Practice by tapping and striking like we did at the end of last lesson by tapping it close and striking it away. Remember to notice the difference at how your hands and arms move when you tap it close and strike it away.*

2B *Now let's start tapping our object into our personal space more up , ahead or down. Remember, hands or arms.*

2C Now start seeing if you can tap it more upward most of the time by keeping the object in your own space by letting it hit the wall, bounce on the ground or come back to you out of the air

2D Let's start playing " Up Tap " see if you can tap your object as often as you can upward by not losing control of it in your space. Remember to go where ever the object goes.

2E Play tap it up this time but on my command use your arms or hands to tap. Make the object go where you want it to go and see how often you can tap it into your space again.

Assessment - Measuring each student tapping his or her object with greater control upward in personal space with desired body parts. (hands and lower arms)

3A Review playing " Up Tap " Remember go where ever the object goes and tap as often as you can. Keep your eye on the object and tap. Are your hands and lower arms tapping your object?

3B Let's play " Tap Count " Count how many total taps you can do before I say stop! Let's try it again and see if you can do more than the first time. Rember go where ever the object goes.

3C With a partner let's play " Partner Tap " . Make your partner a good tapper and feel what it is like to tap it up and soft to your partner and they will tap it back. You might catch it and tap it or just tap it back.

3D Switch to a new partner and make that partner a good tapper like your first partner. Remember! Go where ever the object goes and keep it in your play space.

Assessment – Measuring each student tapping his/ her ball cooperatively to a partner upward with hands or lower arms in personal play space.

Grade Two Lessons

Volley tapping with Your Hands and arms to Yourself and to a Partner.

Second Grade Hand Striking

· ·

Equipment - Lite Weight inflatable Balls, Balloons and taped wrapped balloons for the movement needs of tracking and tapping at a more controlled speed.

Objective – Each student will tap their ball or balloon with greater control in an upward motion with an open hand or hands to self and partner(s).

Body - strike with open hand to self in air , wall, or floor.

Space – Strike in personal space

Effort – strike at low to moderate speeds

Relationship – wall , floor, partner

· ·

Note: The word "volley" is introduced as a movement phrase describing continual tapping/ striking.

1A Play " Up Tap " to yourself by maintaining control in your own space. Remember! Hand back and tap with an open hand under and behind to ball to make in go upward. Keep a controlled speed. Tap your object into the air, at the wall or letting it bounce on the floor.

1B Start to play " Up VolleyTap " by moving where ever the object goes. If your control is really good then tap your object up by making your body move a little more to where you tap your ball. Remember go where ever the ball /object goes.

1C Let's continue playing, but this time let's start to bend our knees to get under the object a little more.

1D Keep playing " Up Volley Tap " but count your taps when you feel ready and see how many you can achieve before I say stop. (2 min.) Remember! Contact your ball with an open hand under and behind the ball. Bend those knees a bit and Tap It! Don't slap it.

1E Let's play " Up Tap " again for 2 min. and compare your score to the first 2 min. challenge of counting. Did your score increase, stay the same or decrease.

Assessment – Measuring each student moving where the object goes by bringing hand and arm back and tapping the object upward with an open hand more often

2A Let's do a 2min. tap challenge like last lesson. See how many taps you can achieve. Remember hand and arm back and tap upward with an open hand and bend those knees.

2B Pair up with a partner and let's play " Partner Tap". Get a rope or a space strip and tap up over the strip to your partner. Try to tap the ball at an easy speed so your partner can tap it back you at an easy speed. Remember! Body ready…Hand back and tap up over the strip.

2C With your partner this time, try to tap your object more as it bounces or out of the air. If you catch and tap back it is OK , but when you feel you can, feel what it is like to tap it back more little often to your partner without catching it.

2D Find a new partner and attempt to tap the object much of the time. Remember to go where ever the object goes and tap it up. Do you feel yourself tapping it more. Are you getting under and behind it?

Assessment – Measuring each student tapping the ball up more often to themselves and to a partner over a low obstacle.

3A Warm –up by playing " Wall Ball " . Have the wall be your partner and play up tap making the object go forward and up at the wall and move to where it goes and continue to volley tap it at the wall. Make sure your hand and arm go back and contact the object behind and under it and bend those knees. (Note: Many Students will usually favor a choice of a ball over a balloon for this developmental task.

3B Now this time see if you can play " Wall Ball " by counting how many total taps you can achieve in 2 min.

3C Let's try it again for 2 min. and see if you can increase your achievement .

3D Pair up with a partner and tap it up and forward so your partner can get it back to you. When you feel that you and your partner have enough tapping control, start counting your taps. See what your achievement is by the time we stop.

3E Find a new partner and see what number of taps you can achieve this time. Remember! It's a tap not a slap.

> **Assessment – Measuring each students frequency in the amount of volley taps they achieve to themselves and to a partner. Arm and hand more consistently goes back and forward and up for contact of object. Knees bending.**

4A Review " Wall Ball " and see how successful you are at tapping at the wall and moving where ever the ball goes. Make sure your hand is back and coming forward , contacting behind and underneath the ball. How was your achievement number this time?

4B Find a partner and play " Partner Wall Ball " . Tap your ball up to the wall so your partner can tap it back to you. Make sure it is a tap not a slap and keep your eye on the ball.

4C Find a new partner and review. Try to make your partner the best tapper they can be and see how often you can keep your taps going. Try to make the ball go where you want it to go and have good control

4E Now choose either " Partner tap over and obstacle or Partner Wall Ball " with your partner. Remember it is a controlled volley tap not a slap and move wherever the object goes and try to volley tap it back.

> **Assessment – Measuring students exploring controlled upward taps by relating to a partner , obstacle, and wall space using desire motion.**

3rd Grade

Volley with Hands and/or Forearms.
(Volleyball like)

. . . .

Equipment - Lite weight inflatable balls, beachballs, Balloons and tape wrapped balloons .

Objective – students will demonstrate volley ball like movements by tracking contacting the object with hands and forearms.

Body – Striking upward with hands and forearms to floor wall and partner.

Relationship – To partner

Space – wall or court space

Effort – Volleying at a controlled speed

. . . .

1A Play " Up Tap " independently . Bend your knees, get hand or hands under and tap up. Feel what it is like to tap in control more often and continually. Remember! You can tap your object up at the wall, air or let it bounce to the floor and tap it up.

1B As you play " Up Tap " add the skill of putting your forearm or forearms out straight and away and extending your arms out ahead of you at your stomach area and attempt to tap the object up with your forearm or forearms at the same time.

Remember to keep those knees bent to get your arms under the object.

1C . As you continue to play " Up Tap " if you tap with your forearms , make sure they are straight and under the object. A balloon can be tapped out of the air and ball on the bounce or in the air.

1D Let's play " Tap Count " . Count how many taps you can achieve in 2 min. with hands or forearms.

1E Let's try it again for another 2 min. and compare your achievement score to the first 2 min.

Assessment – Measuring each student volley taps object upward bending the knees and bumping the ball with greater frequency and proper mechanics.

2A After practicing " Up Tap your own object , let's warm-up by playing " Up Tap " to your partner over a low object. See if you can tap up to your partner by tapping it with your forearm or forearms or tapping it with one or two open hands upward as often as you can. Remember! Knees bent, tap up. (Note; students should have a choice of one forearm or two)

2B Continue tapping and once your consistently tapping with more control, play tap count with your partner and see how many total taps you can do before I say stop. Remember to move wherever the object goes knees bent and tap up with forearm or hands.

2C Find a new partner and see what your tapping achievement is this time before I say stop.

2D With the same partner you have, change your challenge. This time see how many taps you can achieve in a row before losing control and see what your highest in a row total was before I say stop. Remember to extend those arms outward.

2E Repeat your challenge in the same amount of time and see what your in a row achievement is compared to the first challenge.

> *Assessment – Measuring each students ability to continue to tap the object upward over a low obstacle to a partner with knees bent by tapping with forearms or forearms together or open hand taps .*

3A After your " Up Tap " individual warm- up, (this can involve counting taps individuals choose to) find a partner and start tapping over low object. Are your taps gaining in number from last time? Remember, knees bent and hands or forearms under the object as you tap up.

3B Let's play a tapping challenge called " Up and Over ". Start tapping up to your partner over your low obstacle. Remember, move where ever the object goes and tap up to your partner. As soon as you achieve a certain number of taps as a partnership (*this can be a challenging number the students pursue or a number set by the teacher*) add slightly higher obstacle to tap over. (*this can be a cone or plastic bowling pin as an example*).

3C Now that you have achieved a slightly higher obstacle, see if you can achieve a higher challenging achievement goal and when you get their add another obstacle to your "

Up and Over " challenge. (this could be a cone on top off a cone or a pin on top of a cone cone as an example) **Note: The environment is be change for greater challenge.**

3D Find a new partner and start from scratch with a low obstacle and see if you can achieve the same number of obstacles as before. Remember! Knees bent and volley tap up.

> **Assessment - Measuring each student tapping up cooperatively to a partner with greater frequency and challenge themselves by tapping over progressively higher objects by consistently contacting objects with forearms(s) and/**

Volleying Skills Basic to Low Net and Wall Games

3rd Grade

Hand Tennis/ Hand Ball

Note: These skills compliment and transfer inter-task to those skills basic the forehand in: handball, racketball, tennis, squash, badminton as examples.

· ·

Objective – demonstrate volleying skills by contacting object with hands in a volleying motion that is basic to forehand striking.

Equipment – Bouncy inflatable plastics balls of different sizes for differentia

*Body – tapping with an open hand in a forward and upward motion

Space - Personal Play Space at wall or over obstacle

Effort – tapping at a controlled speed

Relationship – to partner , over obstacles, at a wall.

. . . .

1A Play ball tap warm –up on the bounce in your space or at the wall. Try to keep a stiff wrist and open hand. Arm is straight, going back , coming through and tapping the ball forward and up.

1B Continue your practice with the same motion but remember to bend your knees to get under and behind the ball with your hand .

1C This time let's all play " Wall Tap " . Find a medium distance from the wall so your ball can bounce back to you. Let your ball bounce next to you and try to contact it with an open hand behind and under it a bit to make it go forward and up. Remember! Stiff arm back, bend your knees and contact through.

1D Continue tapping and remember to go wherever the ball goes. Make sure now that wherever the ball goes you are tapping it on the bounce and get your body next to it.

1E This time keep tapping and let's play " Tap Count " . Count how many taps you can do before I say stop. Don't forget to keep an open hand and a stiff wrist.

1F Let's try it for the same amount of time again and compare your achievement score. Did it go up?

Assessment – students demonstrate tapping with a stiff wrist and straight swing back and through and knees bent.

2A After you warm –up with " Wall Tap " find a partner and start playing " Hand Tap " with your partner over the tapping strip. Always try to tap the ball on the bounce to your partner he or she can tap it on the bounce back to you. Remember.... Wherever the ball goes you go. Hand back...bend your knees and volley tap through.

2B Continue to tap with your partner and count how many continuous taps you can achieve without losing control. See what your highest achievement number is in 2 min.

2C Try it again for 2 min. and see how your achievement number compares to the first time. Did your number increase?

2D You may want to make your partner move a bit by trying to place the ball into a spot where he or she has to move a bit to tap the ball back to you. Remember, go where the ball goes, bend knees, straight arm back, tap up and through with a stiff wrist and open hand.

2E Find a new partner see if you can make your partner even better than your last partner and see if you can even achieve more taps. Remember! Where ever the ball goes, you go and tap up and forward.

Assessment – Measuring each student consistently demonstrating a "volley tap" to partner in a forehand motion by bend knees at times over a small obstacle.

3A After warming up with wall tap, think if your taps are happening more and more every time you warm up. Are you moving where ever the ball bounces and taping it up and forward.

3B Let's play " Hand Tennis ". Like before, get a strip and tap over the strip with your partner cooperatively and make them move a bit if you feel you have control of your taps.

3C Now it is time to increase our challenge. When you achieve a certain number of taps, add a higher obstacle to tap over. **(As mentioned earlier , numbers of taps can be set by the teacher or students provided the total they are trying to achieve is challenging enough to show skill improvement and obstacles may include cones, plastic bowling pins, chairs, hurdles as an example of obstacles that increase in height**).

3D Let's start our " Hand Tennis " challenge from the beginning with a new partner and see how many obstacles of height that you progress to this time.

Assessment – Measuring each student continuing to tap in a basic forehand motion with greater frequency over increased obstacles of height while playing cooperatively with a partner.

Hand Ball/Wall Ball

Grade 3

· ·

Equipment - Bouncy inflatable bouncy balls of different sizes for differentiation

Body – striking with an open hand

Space – Moderate size personal floor and wall space.

Effort – Applying controlled speed over the ball

Relationship – To partner, floor space and wall space.

Objective – To receive a ball off the wall and in a basic forehand motion " volley tap " the ball to the wall with increased frequency individually and in a partnership.

· ·

1A Let's play " Wall Ball " and tap your ball with and open hand forward and upward to the wall as often as you can. Remember, Straight arm back , bend knees and tap with your arm coming through with a stiff wrist.

1B As you tap , try to move to where ever the ball goes and position yourself next to the ball as you prepare to tap it.

1C As you tap the ball this time concentrate on arm back .....bend knees .....open hand ... tap through

1D Every time you tap , move quickly to wherever the ball goes ...get next to it and tap through.

1E As you tap, see how many taps you can achieve in a given time. Now try again for the same amount of time again and compare your achievement to the first time.

Assessment - students "volley tap " in a basic fore- hand motion at wall tapping the ball with greater consistancy as they receive it on the bounce by moving wherever the ball goes.

2A After your warm – up with ball reflect. Was your ...arm back and straight ....knees bent and tap through with an open hand?

2B This time when you play " Wall Ball " make sure that arm is back and knees as the ball bounces to you. Always try to get next to the ball as you straighten your arm and tap it.

2C Count your achievement of hits and compare your sum total to last time you counted.

2D Now that you have been tapping your ball to the wall , find a partner and play wall tap, tapping your ball up and forward to the wall so it can bounce off the wall and your partner can attempt to tap it on the bounce back to the wall so you can get it.

2E As you tap with your partner more and more try to place your taps into a spot so your partner can get to it one the bounce and tap it back to you, Make your partner the best they can be.

2F When you feel you are both ready, count how many taps you can achieve together before I say stop. Remember, try to get next to the ball and tap it up and forward to the wall.

2E Find a new partner and see what your " Volley Tap " achievement in number of hits is. If it has improved, reflect? What did you do to be better with this partner? Did you move more? Where did you place the ball to your partner.

> ***Assessment - 'Volley Tapping" the ball in a basic forehand motion with greater consistency at the wall with a partner.***

Volleying with Hands Overhead and Forearms (Volleyball Like) in partners and in small groups.

Grade 4

. . . .

Objective – To develop the skill of bumping and setting with proper arm, hand and body position with increased frequency to a partner or partners.

Equipment - Plastic Inflatable balls, Beach Balls.

Body – volleying upward with forearm(s) and hands

Space – personal play/court space

Effort – volleying at a controllable speed.

Relationships – to obstacles, partners and small groups

. . . .

1A Volley your ball by tapping it upward in your own space as often as you can with either a forearm or both forearms at the same time or open hands together or separate with open hands above your head.

1B Now concentrate just on your forearms and try to volley your ball as often as you can. What we are doing is called a " ***Bump*** ". Extend your arms straight out ahead of your waist and wrap one hand around the other to connect your arms and contact your ball as often as you can. Remember. Bend your Knees as you get your forearms under the ball and go wherever the ball goes as you contact it.

1C Now this time as you contact the ball on your forearms , bend and raise those knees a little when contacting the ball. Contact it on your lower forearms as often as you can.

1D Play " Volley Count " and see how many volleys you can make by getting you forearms under the ball. You might let it bounce or volley it out of the air. Remember, Get your forearms straight out away from your body.

1E Now choose a wall space or regular personal space to bump it up to yourself out of the air, on the bounce or at a wall space. Remember, always get those forearms under the ball and bump it upward.

1F Find a partner and play " volley bump". In a personal play space over a low obstacle, try to bump your ball as you receive it on the bounce or in the air up to your partner so that he or she can return it in control back to you.

Assessment - students demonstrate volley contact with a bump by bending knees slightly and connecting arms out straight at stomach level.

2A This time begin to use your open hands to volley when the ball is over your head coming down to you. Look upward at the ball ...place both open hands in front of your eyes and spread your fingers out so you can see through your fingers... when the ball touches your hands tap the ball upward with your fingers and hands.

2B Now play " Up Volley Tap " to yourself by trying to contact the ball on your forearms when it comes down below your head and try to push a tap upward when you contact it above your head.

2C Continue tapping both ways as often as you can remember to bend those knees to allow your body to get more under the ball.

2D This time as you spread your fingers to see through them , make a window with you thumbs and fore fingers touching so it looks like a triangle you can see through. What we are doing is called a " **Set** " . When the ball comes down to your hands , just like before , push upward with your fingers and hands as you contact the ball.

2E Now this time set and bump as often as you can. Remember, get your forearms and hands under the ball and bend your knees. Go where ever the ball goes. Use a **bump and set when** you feel you have to. (**Note: *there will be times when students will react with one arm bumps and one hand taps . This is not discouraged, but viewed as necessary on a path to greater object control as the begin to develop for frequency in their bump** and **sets***

2F Play " Tap Count " and count how many volleys you can achieve by bumping and setting.

3A After warming up with your bumps and sets in your own space and see how often you can volley it directly from the air.

3B Now go to a wall space and practice your bumps at a wall by always making your ball bump upward and rebound back to you.

3C This time as you do your wall bumps see how often you can contact your ball out of the air as it rebounds back from the wall.

3D Find a partner and a rope or space strip to put on the floor to volley over to your partner. Again, make your partner the best he or she can be by bumping your ball back and forth to your partner up and over the obstacle you have on the floor. Remember, bend your knees to get your forearms under the ball as you contact.

3E Play " tap count " and count how many bumps you and your partner can achieve before I say stop.

3F Find a new partner and see what your " tap count " achievement is before I say stop.

> **Assessment – Measuring proper bumping mechanics with arms straight and knees bent volleying to partner with frequency.**

4A After you warm up with your own personal bumps and sets to yourself. Find a partner and a low obstacle and see how often you" bump it when you can" and "set it " when you can up and over to your partner.

4B Keep bumping and setting to your partner but now see how often the ball never hits the ground.

4C Think of every bump and set as a pass to your partner that makes your partner good at bumping and setting the ball out of the air and back to you.

Remember if you are bumping or setting to get under the ball by bending you knees.

4D Let's play " Keep it Up " and see how many times you can keep the ball up to you partner by bumping and setting the ball over your obstacle so you partner can get it back to you. Try to get the most you have ever achieved.

4E Now switch to a new partner and see what your achievement is.

> **Assessment – measuring student ability to bump and set to partner with proper mechanics and an emphasis on frequency.**

5A After your individual warm up of bumping and setting to yourself, form a group of three and have one person bump and set across the obstacle to 2 people. The side with two people will decide who contacts the ball as it travels over the obstacle so he or she can bump or set it back to the one person on the other side.

5B Once you have it down, see if you can play " Keep it Up " in a group three by trying to place the ball in an area that the person across the obstacle can receive by bumping setting or tapping it back to the other 2 people. Count your achievement.

5C After a while rotate positions so that over time each person has a chance to be individually on one side of the obstacle and next to a partner on the other side.

5E Form a new group of three and repeat your " Keep it Up" challenge and see what your achievement is this time.

Assessment – Measuring proper bumping and setting mechanics and the basic understanding of passing.

6A At the conclusion of your bump and set warm up (as students become more competent and mature in their volleying skills , the warmup can include a partner) form a group of four and function as a cooperative team with 2 people on each side of the obstacle trying to play " Keep it Up " to the other 2 people.

6B Begin to call for the ball if it comes to your space and tap, bump or set it over so that one of the other players can return it back to your side. Remember..... Knees bent and make sure you are under the ball to tap, set or bump it up and over to the other team.

6C Play " Keep it Up " as a team of four trying to make your partners across the obstacle the best players they can be by tapping, bumping or setting to their spaces so they can receive the ball by volleying it back to you.6D Start to count and see what your achievement score is as a team of four. Try again and see if you can achieve a greater number than the first time for the same time period.

6E Form a new group of four and repeat your challenge as a team and see what your achievement is.

Assessment – Measuring proper bumping and setting mechanics across obstacle to a small group and basic understanding of spacial tactics.

Hand Tennis Grade Four

Note: This unit compliments and can transfer positively to those skills common to forehand motions related to handball, racket ball, tennis, squash , badminton and others not mentioned.

* *

Equipment - Small to moderate sized plastic inflatable balls, bouncy foam balls.

Body – striking with and open hand, straight arm in an upward, with a back to forward motion.

Space - moderate sized personal floor space

Effort – providing controlled speed over ball

Relationship – to partner, group and obstacles.

* *

1A After your individual warm up find a partner and review tapping over an obstacle of low height (such as a cone or bowling pin) and keeping it in play on the other side of your partner's court so he or she can return it back to you. "Remember …Open hand …stiff wrist …arm back and follow through ".

1B As you begin to increase your number of volleys to your partner, start to increase the height of your obstacle that you volley over. Set a goal of number of volleys where your control gets better and once you achieve that number increase the height of your obstacle a bit (Again his can be an elementary chair or an elementary hurdle as example)

1C Now it's time to increase your challenge by forming a group of four with 2 players on each side of the obstacle you've placed. Make sure it is moderate to low height and adjust the right height to how much volleying control your doubles group has.

1D As you volley across the side to the other side of the court make sure that you begin to communicate to your partner . Phrases like " I've got it! It's mine !" are good phrases to use.

1E Play tap count in doubles. How many taps can your doubles groups achieve in a certain amount of time. Try it for the same time again and see what your achievement is.

1F Find a new group of four or just a new partnership with the partner you have and repeat the same challenge.

Volleying with Rackets /Paddles

Areas of Movement

● ●

Body – Striking object with a paddle / racket on the face of it from different areas of the body.

Space - Personal,General , high medium and low

Effort – Striking an object at different speeds and force.

Relationship – to manipulatives (racket/paddles), obstacles and other students.

● ●

Grade One

Striking Balloons or small beach balls with a Paddle

Objective - that each student track and tap his or her balloon with greater frequency on the face of the paddle individually and to a partner.

1A Find a paddle and a balloon. Hold your paddle with your strong hand on the handle like you are shaking it's hand. Remember to wrap your hand around the handle and grip it so you are holding on to it. Try to tap your balloon or beach ball on the big flat part paddle as often as you can. We call that the face of the paddle.

1B You can tap it from the ground, or from the air or from your hand. You can give it a good tap but don't smash it.

1C Keep tapping the object. Can you feel the face of the paddle always contacting your object?

1D Now begin tapping your balloon or beach more often and attempt to always tap it with the face of your paddle. Remember! Keep your eye on the ball and where ever you tap the balloon or beach ball, go where it goes and continue trying to tap it.

1E Let's tap from different areas of our body. Demonstrate an over hand swing, both side arm swings, (**commonly referred to at more mature levels of skill as the " Forehand, Backhand and Over hand**) one side and the other side and an under-hand swing or overhand swing. Now begin to tap your balloon or beach ball from these areas of your body when the

have to and see how often you can continue to tap. Think...
What area of your body are you taping from right now?

1F Let's now tap from these areas when you hear my command." Tap overhand "...Tap from one side.....Now tap from the other side ....Now tap from under hand". Remember! Where ever the balloon or beach ball goes you go."

1G Let's play " Keep it Up Count Tap " . Count how many taps you can without letting the balloon touch the ground until I say stop Let's try it again to see if our achievement may improve.

> ***Assessment – can each student with greater frequency tap the object with face of the paddle consistently from ground and or air.***

2A Warm up by yourself with your balloon or beach ball and paddle and remember to tap from those different areas of your body from the last lesson.

2B Let's add the challenge and let's review " Tap Count" to my command and finish when I say stop .Tap overhand..... side arm ...other side.... and underhand. L

2C Find a partner with a tapping strip or rope to hit over. Tap the balloon or beach to your partner and as the balloon or beach ball comes back to you, try to tap it directly back to your partner. See how often you can keep it going.. and remember that you can tap it from the ground or from the air.

2D Find a new partner and see how well you keep it going. Count if you like and see what you achievement can be. **(Keeping counts optional is appropriate to not overload those** students who need to focus more on the movement and relationship to the paddle and balloon.)

Assessment – measuring each student's ability to track the balloon or beach ball from the ground or air and tap it with increased frequency on the face of the paddle individually and to a partner cooperatively.

3A Find a balloon or beach ball and this time play " Off the Ground". Your goal is to tap your object with the face of the paddle up into the air as often as you can. Remember, eye on ball and go where ever ball goes and always contact on the face of the paddle.

3B Let's play "Tap Count". Count how many taps you can make that don't touch the ground. (**encourage students to choose an object that gives them increased control. Balloons may be chosen more often because of the challenge of tracking in the air and volleying**).

3C Let's try again, but this time listen to my command. Overhead, Side, Underhand. How did you achieve this time? Did you have to move your feet more often?

3D Let's find a partner and play off the ground over a tapping strip. Make your partner the best player he or she can be tapping your balloon up to your partner so he or she can tap it back to you. Move your feet to go wherever the object goes …eye on object and tap up.

3E With your partner play "Off the Ground " see how often you can tap so it doesn't touch the ground. Remember...Tap the object back to your partner up and over your floor strip.

3F Find new partner and see how successful you can be this time (**Again, depending on how the successful each partnership is, quantifying volleys can be an option because some partnerships may need to just focus on tracking and volleying successfully**).

Assessment – measuring each students ability to track out of the air and tap on the face of the paddle individually and in a partnership with greater frequency.

Grade Two

Volleying with Paddles and Balloons Individually and in Partnerships over obstacles.

Objective – that each student taps with increased frequency individually and to a partner from different areas of the body over.

1A Find a paddle and balloon of your choice and warm up by volleying from different areas of your body ..overhand , strong side ... other side.... and underhand. Remember to try to keep the balloon from hitting the ground.

1B Play a quick challenge of " Tap Count Keep it Up ". Finish when I say stop.

1C Find a partner and directly tap over your tapping strip to your partner. Play " Keep it Up" . *Remember to go where the balloon goes and tap it from that area of your body on the face of your paddle that gets the balloon back to your partner. Make sure your paddle is prepared to volley tap.*

1D Play " Tap Count Keep it up " and see what you can achieve before I say stop. Let's try it a second time for the same amount of time and see if we improved. Remember it is a tap not a smash.

1E Let's now move to volleying over a higher obstacle. When you achieve number of volley taps that I have set for us, you will get a cone to volley tap over to your partner.

Assessment - Measuring how often the paddle contacts the object in flight.

2A After practicing your taps from different areas of your body individually, find a partner and volley tap over your strip in good control . Remember it is a volley tap not a smash.

2B Again when you when you achieve the number of volley taps between you and your partner that I have set for the class get a cone to hit over. **(the goal may be adjust higher for greater challenge and success)**

2C Now you and your partner set a goal that you can achieve but challenging enough to improve. Once you achieve that goal, add another obstacle to make it a little higher for greater challenge. (some examples could be a chair, stool or larger cone).

2D Find a new partner and practice at the obstacle level you are at. Set a goal. When you achieve your new goal, add another obstacle to get a little higher. (adding cones to cones or cones to chairs/stools is always a way to increase height somewhat).

> *Assessment - Measuring the ability to volley the object with the paddle at greater height cooperatively with a partner..*

Grade Three

Volleying with Paddles with Balloons of varying sizes and light foam balls individually and in partnerships.

Objective – For each student to volley from different areas of the body with a beginning emphasis of forehand and back hand motion cooperatively with a partner.

1A Choose either a small, medium or large balloon to volley with from different areas of the body individually, Over hand ….. forehand …..backhand (**which was referred to grade 1 and 2 as one side and the other side**) and underhand. Remember it is a volley tap, not a smash.

1B Now that you have tapped from different areas of your body with good control. (**the teacher can certainly choose as an option " Keep it up tap count " for a quantifiable for of measurement as was implemented in grade 1 and 2)** You may choose a foam ball if you like and attempt to tap volley in control. You may add the wall to tap to if you choose and let the ball bounce or volley tap it out of the air.

1C Play " Tap Count " and see what your achievement is when I say stop.

1D Now find a partner and tap over your tapping strip. *Remember ... a smaller balloon is of greater challenge as is a foam ball because they tend to travel a bit faster*. Use the object that gives you control and change it if you need a greater challenge or a lesser to improve. **Remember to have your paddle ready to volley tap.**

1E Play " Tap Count " when you are ready and see what you achievement is when I say stop. Remember! Always keep your eye on the object and volley tap it on the face of the paddle so your partner can get it.

Assessment – measuring students ability to volley from different areas of body with greater frequency.

2A After your volley tap warmup. (**quantifiable form of measurement can be an option**) Find a partner and warmup over your tapping strip with good control using the object of your choice for achievement.

2B Once you have good control, set a goal for yourselves. Once you achieve this goal, get your first obstacle. Remember to make your goal challenging enough for constant improvement. (**quantifiable form of measurement**)

2C Set a second goal. Make that goal more challenging to achieve your second obstacle which is a greater height than the first.

2D Now work at achieving your third goal of greater challenge for your highest obstacle. (**obstacles should usually stay in the moderate range of height**)

2E Find a new partner and count how many taps you can achieve with the obstacles in place. (**a nice option is to play a classroom challenge , where we all add up our scores and see what the class achieved as a whole**)

> *Assessment – measuring students ability to tap with consistency and greater frequency from different areas of the body with slight emphasis on beginnings of forehand backhand motion.*

Grade Four

Volleying with a Paddle or Short Racket with small balloons, foam balls or big badminton birdies. Introduction of forehand and backhand skills.

. . . .

> *Body - striking with a racket/paddle.*

> *Space - Moderate size personal floor and wall space.*

> *Effort – striking at a controlled speed*

> *Relationship – partners, obstacles, walls , small groups*

. . . .

1A Choose and object of your choice and begin to volley it in control with your short paddle or racket. Volley tap it up ....

or at the wall...or one the bounce. Choose the object that gives you control.

1B Now concentrate at using different areas of your body to tap from. Back hand....forehand....underhand... overhand. Get your paddle/racket ready each time you prepare to tap. Play "volley tap count ". Chart your achievement when I say stop.

1C Find a partner and choose a strip to tap over. Remember.... paddle ready and volley tap over. Keep your paddle ready and tap from the area of your body you must when the object comes to you. Remember to choose the object that gives you control.

1D Play " Volley Tap Count " when you achieve the goal you set, get a higher object each time. Remember to make your goal challenging and successful so you can keep moving forward.

Assessment - measuring the frequency of the arm crossing body and moving backward in backhand and arm moving back from strong side in forehand.

2A After your warm-up with the object of your choice, find only a bouncing foam ball and play "bounce tap" by tapping your ball up in your space and letting it drop to the ground and bounce up and tapping it up to yourself each time on each bounce.

2B Now concentrate on your forehand from your strong side and continue to tap your ball up. Paddle/Racket back ......

come through and tap up. Make your paddle/racket get under the ball and continue to tap.

2C Now start to bend your knees a little if you need to make sure your paddle/racket is under the ball as you tap each time.

2D Begin practicing wall ball with a bouncing foam ball. "Volley tap"the ball to the wall and retrieve it on the bounce by volley tapping it back and up each time. Go where ever the ball goes and try to volley tap a forehand from you strong side.

2E Now try to always volley tap with the side of your body facing the wall if you can.

2F Once you feel you have some control, play 'volley tap count " and see what you can achieve.. Try it again and see if you can achieve more when I say stop.

> ***Assessment – Measuring the ability to position side of body at times and with proper arm/paddle motion. Slight emphasis of knee bend.***

3A After your warm-up with your forehand. Find a partner and begin to play wall ball and try to always tap to your partner's strong side. When gain the control you want see how many you can achieve. Remember! Paddle/ racket back .... Tap through and up a bit.

3B Find a new partner and try the same challenge. Remember to bend your knees if you need to get under the ball a bit.

3C With you new partner see how many in a row you can achieve. Try it again and see you if achieve more.

> ***Assessment - Measuring basic forehand (strong side) mechanics. Paddle/Racket coming through , forward and up and ready position.***

4A During your warm up, focus your taps on your strong side "forehand" and your other side " backhand " with a balloon to volley tap in the air or a foam ball to volley tap at the wall and back to you. As the ball or balloon comes to you, try to respond by tapping it from your strong side or your other side

4B Now begin to think of putting your body in the correct position to contact the ball from your forehand or backhand by adjusting what side of your hips face the direction you are volleying to by positioning your feet to face the side of your body in that direction. Quickly...when the balloon or ball approaches ...move your feet in that position and volley.

4C Once you are in position, try to bring your paddle back and volley through, Remember! It is a volley, not a smash.

4D Now as you volley, think of these words Ready position! .....paddle back ....volley through. Remember! Trying to keep your volley motion forward and a bit upward when you volley through. When you feel ready to count play " Volley Tap Count ". When I say stop. Chart your achievement. Let's try again for the same amount of time. How did you do this time?

> ***Assessment - Measuring " side ready " body position to receive ball and paddle back and coming through.***

5A Warmup with your forehand and back hand and remember your body position and the volleying cues from last lesson. Ready position!....Paddle back....Volley through.

5B Find a partner and either at the wall with a ball or over a floor strip with a balloon try to volley to your partner by focusing on volleys from your forehand and back hand. Make your partner a great player by trying to give he or she a volley that can be returned each time.

5C Find a new partner and continue. If you are hitting over a floor strip, set a goal to achievement a higher obstacle such as a cone or a small chair. Remember! As you volley, through keep you motion forward and a little upward.

5D With your partner play " Volley Tap Count". See what you can achieve when I say stop.

5E Now every partnership will use a floor strip and an obstacle if they choose to volley to their partner with either a bouncy ball or balloon . Remember to react with your forehand or backhand if you have to and get your body ready to volley.

Assessment – measuring ready positions, paddle/racket back , volley through and up, forehand and backhand side. to partner.

Grade Five

Refining forehand and greater development of backhand strokes/volleys.

· ·

Objective – That each student demonstrate a more mature backhand and forehand motion with proper body and foot position as he or she volleys a ball with a paddle/racket.

Equipment – Bouncy foam, inflatable plastic balls of moderate to smaller size or bouncy wiffle balls.

· ·

1A Get a paddle/short racket and a bouncing foam ball (sometimes a **wiffle ball** that bounces works well too) and go to a wall space and practice your forehand volley by remembering to position your feet shoulder width with your opposing side of your body facing the wall. As the ball comes to you......racket/paddle back... arm somewhat parallel to the floor as you volley slightly upward and through. Try to always volley the ball on the bounce back to the wall.

1B Now try to focus on your other side by making your backhand a little stronger remember to position your feet shoulder width , try to extend your arm a little straighter as it crosses your body and you bring it back ready to volley. Like the forehand keep it somewhat parallel and volley through. Try to keep your wrist stiff for control as you contact and volley through.

1C Now practice wall volleys by volleying to your forehand and back hand as you react each time to the ball on the bounce. Think of these words: **forehand**.........ready position.....move feet...paddle/racket back.... volley through... **backhand**...... ready position....move feet.....paddle/racket .....across your body and back.... volley through.

1D Continue volleying to back hand and forehand but now focus on **bending your knees a bit** as you volley through.

1E Play " volley tap count " at the wall and see what your achievement is. Try again for the same period of time and compare your achievement to the first time.

> *Assessment – measuring proper arm and paddle/ racket motion, arm straight back follow through forward and up. Proper foot and body positon prior to swing.*

2A After your warm up at the wall with your forehand and back hand, find a partner and play partner wall ball attempting to react with forehand and back hand volleys off the wall to each other. Remember your body words....feet in position...paddle/racket back...volley through. Remember to parallel your paddle/racket somewhat to ground as you volley through.

2B Play " volley tap count " with your partner and chart your achievement.

2C Now with your partner and a bouncy ball, see if you can play " short court ping pong by volley tapping to your partner across the strip so he or she can receive it on the bounce and volley tap it back. Try to make your partner the best player he or she be by giving a controlled volley as often as you can.

2D Time for our " volley tap count challenge " and chart your achievement until I say stop.

2E Find a new partner and see what your achievement will be this time.

> **Assessment – Measuring ability to receive a ball from the wall or across court from a partner will proper body position, arm and paddle motion form forehand or backhand area.**

3A After your warm up with your forehand and back hand skills, find a partner and review short court volleying with your partner. Choose an obstacle of low to moderate height and remember to volley to allow your partner to volley back on the bounce. Make your partner the best player he or she can be by placing your ball in a spot that they can return a volley with control.

3B Remember the important skill words used in your volley and count how many in a row you and your partner achieve. The more volleys you achieve in a row the control your control will be.

3C Let's move to doubles play. With you making your court space wider, have two people on each side attempt to volley their ball over to a returnable spot on the other court so that one of the two receivers can return a controlled volley back. As we work cooperatively with our group of four begin to communicate your partner and say " I've got it " or" It's Mine " to signal that you will be volleying it over to other court.

3D A good measurement of your communication and volleying control as a doubles group is to see how (volley tap count) many volleys you can achieve before I say stop! Try it again and see what your achievement is this time when I say stop.

3E Let's do an in a row " volley tap count challenge " for greater challenge this time. Set a goal for your doubles group and see what you can achieve before the time period of your challenge is up.

> *Assessment – measuring proper body position and arm and paddle motion in a volley by receiving a ball from a player in the opposing court. Demonstrating positioning in open space with a doubles partner.*

Grade Five

Volleyball Skills

Developing an Underhand Serve and the Introduction to Simple Tactics.

Objective – That each student will demonstrate the correct motion of an underhand serve and begin to develop the skill of proper positioning in open space and attempt to bump or set a volley to a teammate when receiving the ball form the opposing court.

Equipment – Lite volleyball trainers of large to moderate size and moderate size plastic inflatable balls with some tape around for slightly greater weight.

Body – striking with slightly close hand in underhand motion, bumping with forearms and setting with open hands.

Space – larger personal court space.

Effort – volleying at controlled speed to pass or volleying over net.

Relationship – to team, group, and moderate to higher obstacle.

* *

1A Use a light plastic ball or a trainer and practice your" bumps" to yourself or up at a wall to receive the ball back to you each time. When you bump, remember to bend your knees a bit…. Wrap one hand around the other extend your arm outs ahead at stomach height. Try to contact the ball on your forearms each time and volley upward.

1B Now practice over hand " sets" to yourself. Remember bend your knees again……place your hands facing palms toward ceiling , above your face …make a triangle with your forefingers and thumbs connected and contact the ball on your fingers and look through that triangle when volleying each time you are able to set.

1C Keep setting. Try to get those elbows out as you form your triangle and when you contact with your fingers, straighten those arms and push upward.

1D Now as you warm up try to alternate your bumps and sets at times. Remember to bend your knees and get under the ball and contact it upwards.

Score yourself and play " volley tap count " . How many can you do all together before I say stop. Try it a second time and compare your achievement.

1E Find a partner and play" bump and set " to each other. Again, make your partner a great player by trying to give them a bump or set that they can receive. Its ok to volley it on the bounce or in the air. Remember to bend your knees to get under the ball and use a floor strip if you like.

Assessment – Measuring that each student demonstrates correct body, arm hand position before and during bumping and setting volleys.

2A After you review your warm up with your bumps and sets, find a partner and do the same. Count your " volleys " if you like.

2B Now with your partner, attempt to volley your ball as an" underhand server". Place your ball in your opposite hand, out in front of you and bring your strong arm back and contact it out of your holding hand with an underhand motion using a part of your hand. Send it to your partner so they can catch it. Take turns being a catcher and a server. Remember to keep the ball still in your holding hand and use a part of your hand to contact it up and forward to your partner.

2C Now see if you can serve it to your partner so he or she can bump or set it back to you so you can catch it.

2D Let's now play " Keep it Up" in a group of three by attempting to bump and set when it is possible to do so. To start off, use a bump set or serve. Use the one you can control the best. There may be times where a one handed hit has to be done with your forearm or open hand. Make each other the best they can be by always making controlled volleys.

2E What made you successful if you kept the ball going? Think of your body, arms hands and knees. Were they in the right position and where you always getting under the ball?

> *Assessment – Measuring how each student in a group of three demonstrates correct bumping and setting mechanics by moving and positioning body correctly by passing to teammate in the group.*

3A After warming up with individually and with a partner, find a group of four and make a court with a floor strip or rope as you low obstacle. Practice playing 2 with 2 over the obstacle by volleying it on the bounce or in the air. Always try to give the other partners a returnable volley and attempt to bump and set your ball when you can. Like in your group of three , start your ball freely with what gives you control, a serve, bump or set.

> *Assessment – Measuring how each student moves to position him or herself so he or she can bump and set when possible to the opposing court. Also measuring basic mechanics regarding underhand serve and set and more mature mechanics regarding bump. (Knees bent arms extended straight, contact on forearms).*

3B See how well you can keep the ball going back to the opposing court.

3C Now when you feel ready, attempt to pass your ball to your partner by volleying it up to him or her so he or she can volley it over to the opposing court.

3D As you volley it , now try to hit it out of the air more often. See how often your group of four can keep the ball up in the air without it touching the ground.

4A After your volleying warm ups let's make groups of 6's and make your court like last lesson but this time with 3 people to each side playing 3 with 3. Let's start to position ourselves in spaces that give us room to receive a volley from the other court and pass it to a teammate. Make a triangle with 2 in front and none in back or one in front and two in back.

4B Remember start your ball freely with a serve, bump or set. We are playing as a team of six attempting to keep our ball going as often as we can to the opposing court. Try to volley that ball out of the air as often as you can.

4C Play" volley count" and see how often you can keep it going. How successful was your group? What contributed to your success? Did you keep you spaces as positions that didn't interfere with another player.

4D Let's explore playing 3 vs.3 keeping of obstacle as either a floor or coned obstacle. When the ball comes to your side you can volley it up to an open space to the opposing court where other players aren't or attempt to volley it as a teammate as a pass and he or she can volley it to an open court space on the other side.

CHAPTER 6

Activity Based Movement Experiences

Activity based movement experiences involve whole class or large portions of a class participating in a simultaneous activity together in an **open skill environment** with each other with one common goal and a variety of basic tactics. The emphasis is to apply those skills practiced in other developmental movement experiences. Some examples of these activities can be **dodgeball**, **battleship** , **target ball and poison ball** just to name a few. One side sends available objects across to the other side with a goal of sending it to a target, open space or to a person. When implementing an activity, one must always gage if the activity compliments the movement skills being developed, in this case volleying skills and that the tactics and concepts are understood for that age level.

As a note: An activity environment also has more stimuluses to it. Regarding the variety of stimulus that students may be exposed to at the same time can include concepts, tactics rules and changing space. These experiences can be engaging and challenging, but as a result, there may be times that the quality of the skill may lower based on the student's focus on other stimuli. Redirection to a student or students back to proper skill when participating is always recommended.

Volleying Group/Class Activity

● ●

Body – striking with hands and lower arms or racket/paddle

Space – sending the ball consistently to general open space.

Effort – Volleying with various speeds over the object to place it in various parts of the opposing court.

Relationships- to other players and open court space.

● ●

It's important to Note: These activities are appropriate for classes and students who can often track a ball and volley an object with the hand or arm or racket/paddle as a multi-functional volleying activity. Volleying in hand tennis or hand ball like motions and volleyball like motions. Activities tend to provide environments that are less predictable and require a growing understanding of spacial and effort (applying force over and object) concepts that are *dynamic and often involve constant change in those movement areas.* When reading through these activities, you certainly may be aware of other activities not included in this text that you may be familiar with that teach the same skills by a different name or varied concepts. By implementing an activity based teaching approach, these questions are often asked when reflecting on the abilities of students.

1. Do students as a whole often apply volleying skills to their movements when participating in the activity? Can they track the object well?

2. Does the activity maximize each student's participation in applying volleying skills?

3. Are students as a whole capable of applying various levels of force over the object?

4. Can students as a whole apply spacial concepts such as using open space to position themselves and volley the object into apposing spaces.

Knowing the answers to these questions can help the teacher choose an activity that is most appropriate to the developmental needs of the class as a whole and pursue any adaptations if necessary. Listed are 8 activities targeted to enhance the volleying experience in elementary age students. **Note:** Purposeful adaptation is always recommended for the benefit of the differential needs of the students.

"Clear Your Side" (Can also be referred to as " Clear Your Room ")

Divide the gym in half, length wise for larger group sizes within the activity or divide it into two halves width wise for moderate size groups within the activity. This decision should be based on the level of developmental ability of volleying skills in each class. The smaller the group activity the less complexity exists regarding relating to others and using space. The activity in very basic by design and includes a simple goal. **Each student on one side of the gym will attempt to volley any ball he or she sees over to the other side of the gym. The object is to get as many balls out of your team's side and onto the other side of the gym.**

Basic Rules:

1. Always attempt to volley your object into open space to the other side of your play space where the opposing group/team is.

2. Try not to carry and collect balls. Focus on individual balls to volley to the other side.

Adding Manipulatives - Rackets and/or Paddles.

Basic Rules:

1. Use a paddle or racket. When a ball comes to your side, attempt to strike (volley) it with your paddle or racket over to the other side off the ground or from the air into open space.

2. Focus on individual balls and don't collect balls to hit.

Target Ball (added Variation for Challenge)

This activity functions in the same manner as clear your side, but there are placed in a variety of areas on each side of the gym various targets such as pins or cones that students attempt to aim for and hit with the ball they are volleying with. Each student can attempt to protect the target or roam freely though out his or her team's space looking to strike or volley the ball at the opposing teams targets.

Basic Rules:

1. Only one person can guard a target.

2. Once the object is in the target or contacts the target, you can send that object back the opposing team's targets.

Up and Over

The object of this activity is for the students to focus on volleying over objects. Break the class into two halves so the courts are shorter and there are fewer students to each side so there is less complexity and more participation for each student. Divide both courts with cones that serve as obstacles to volley over into the other court. Use balloons or balls to volley with. As the object comes into the court, a team member will attempt to volley the object over to an open court space on the other side. Once again the concept is to volley as many objects as possible to the opposing teams court as a variety of objects are continually in play to maximize participation.

Basic Rules: Explained in Description

Keep It Up/Group Tap/

This activity is more cooperative by design. The group can function with roughly 5 to six students in a circle. With a ball or balloon appropriate for the developmental needs of the group, the object is simply volleyed up on the bounce or in the air and randomly retrieved by another group/team member. The goal is to attempt to keep the object going by volleying continually as a group. This also develops good team communication skills (relationships) and spacial skills.

Basic Rules: Explained in Description

Short Court Clear Away

In groups of 4 to 6 (with four of five balloons being used simultaneously) three people of two people from each side clear in a smaller court space any balloon that comes to their side by volleying it over of floor obstacle of appropriate height for the developmental needs of the students participating. Although this activity is just a smaller group version of clear you side, Students still need to continually react to a balloon coming over to their side of the court and volley it back (forehand, backhand, overhand, underhand) This is a good lead up to a larger class activity like "Clear Your Side " because of less complexity and fewer objects and students to relate to. You can adaptive the activity for paddles and rackets.

Basic Rules: Explained in Description

Circle Pass/ Cooperative Volley

This activity relates more to hand tennis/hand ball skills *almost like and "Upward four Square "*. Being cooperatively based, groups of four, six or eight form a circle. Using one ball for the group each player taps the ball upward and on the bounce to another player within the circle, so that player will react with an upward controlled volley on the bounce to another player. The emphasis is on being in a ready position. As the activity becomes more advanced communication is encouraged. The activity could be adapted for a greater challenge by adding 2 balls simultaneously.

Basic Rules: Explained in description

Circle Paddle/ Cooperative Volley

Cooperatively based, Groups of four or six form a circle and like "Keep It Up " one larger sized balloon is used for each student to tap about the circle to another group member and react to the balloon and tap it from the appropriate area of the body (forehand side, backhand side, underhand and overhand). Again positions of readiness and communication are emphasized and once again an added challenge could be 2 balloons simultaneously.

Basic Rules: Explained in description.

Volcano Volley

This activity basically falls in line with building the volleying process of the lesson by learning to volley over obstacles of increased height. The goal is to do whatever you can to keep the object you are volleying over off the volcano lava. In this case is the ground or your floor obstacle. When you become more successful at volleying, by the increase number of volleys, whether in a row or collective you can begin to grow your volcano with higher floor obstacles. Raising these obstacles can function as a meaningful motivator for students to achieve greater benchmarks in their abilities to volley over objects of greater height.

Basic Rules : Explained in Description

Reflecting By Looking at the Whole Picture

Through these processes of learning, What Can We Accomplish? Reflecting back on *Physical Literacy*, we can observe that through the findings, that those who move well in a variety of ways tend to be more active through their childhood and adult years, leading to healthier lifestyles. This book has targeted one form of *Physical Literacy* as a guide to a process that enhances success and keeps our students moving forward in their abilities as successful movers as they encounter various challenges in the area of volleying games (net and wall games) , activities and sports. Whatever movement experiences students choose it is my wish , and hopefully the wish of any Physical Educator that their choice is based on success, purpose and fun.

REFERENCES

Abels, Karen W., Bridges Jennifer M. (2010) Teaching Movement Education, Human Kinetics

Rink, Judith H. (2014) Seventh Addition Teaching Physical Education for Learning, McGraw Hill

(2017) Coach Ireland , Physical Literacy

Logsdon, Bette J. , Alleman Luann M., Straits Sue Ann, Belka David E., Clark Dawn (1997) Second Edition, Physical Education Unit Plans for Grades 1 – 2, Human Kinetics

Logsdon Bette J., Alleman Luann M., Straits Sue Ann, Belka David E., Clark Dawn (1997) Second Edition , Physical Education Unit Plans for Grades 3 – 4 ,Human Kinetics

Logsdon Bette J., Alleman Luann M., Straits Sue Ann, Belka David E., Clark Dawn (1997) Second Edition , Physical Education Unit Plans for Grades 5 – 6 ,Human Kinetics

Ward Phillip, Lewald Harry (2018) Effective Physical Education and Instruction *An Evidence Based and Teacher tested Approach* , page 446

Landy Joanne M., Landy Maxwell J., (1992) Ready to Use P.E. Activities Grades 3 – 4, Parker Publishing Company

Scheimer Suzann (1999) Assessment Strategies for Elementary Physical Education, Human Kinetics

USA School Tennis Curriculum *A Step-by-Step Guide to Teaching Tennis in Schools* Eighth Edition (2000) United States Tennis Association

Shape America National Standards & Grade Level Outcomes for K - 12 Physical Education (2014) Human Kinetics

Kamiya Artie (2017) *Cooperative Volleying* http//sports video.com You Tube

ABOUT THE AUTHOR

Dave Olszewski has taught for over 30 years Elementary Physical Education in New Hampshire. He recently received the 2017 New Hampshire Elementary Physical Education Teacher of The Year Award and teaches part time at New England College as a Professor in the Kinesiology Department. He is past President of NHAPHERD and has served on the New Hampshire State Arts Frameworks Board as a Physical Education Representative in the area of Dance in the 1990's.